Healthy Mama, Healthy Baby.

Your guide to achieving optimum health after delivery.

By

Paul Esther Innocent

Table of Content

Introduction

Mothers carry part of their baby with them forever in their heart and sometimes with souvenirs on their body. You have just been through a life changing experience. Having a baby touches your mind, body, and spirit. You may feel differently about yourself and the world. This is a time to honor the experience you've just had and take good care of yourself.

People often talk about how to care for a baby once he or she is born. However, they do not often talk about what mothers may experience after giving birth. New mothers often have many questions about their bodies and emotions.The problems and discomforts a woman experiences after having a baby are not often talked about.This doesn't mean that they are not common.

It's okay to feel worried about these symptoms and to get advice about how to deal with them.
This book will give you insight and guide you to taking practical steps to ensure better health for you and in turn, your baby.

Chapter 1

What is postpartum care?

The postpartum period refers to the first six weeks after childbirth. This is a joyous time, but it's also a period of adjustment and healing for mothers. During these weeks, you'll bond with your baby and you'll have a post-delivery checkup with your doctor.

The 6 weeks after pregnancy and delivery of a baby is when the mother's body returns to its pre-pregnancy state.

After childbirth, a mother can expect to have some physical changes and symptoms, but they are usually mild and temporary. Severe health issues are rare.

Caring for a new baby while feeling sore, tired and stressed can be a lot to handle. Taking care of yourself is one of the best things you can do for your baby.
Many things are happening in your body right after you have a baby. During pregnancy, your body changed a lot. It worked hard to keep your baby safe and healthy. Now that your baby is here, your body is changing again. Some of these changes are physical, like your breasts getting full of milk. Others are emotional, like feeling extra stress.

Many discomforts and body changes after giving birth are normal. But sometimes they're signs or symptoms of a health problem that needs treatment. Go to all of your postpartum checkups, even if you're feeling fine. These are medical checkups you get after having a baby to make sure

you're recovering well from labor and birth.
The most common complications after childbirth are the following:

- Excessive bleeding (postpartum hemorrhage)
- Infections of the uterus
- Bladder and kidney infections
- Breast infection
- Problems with breastfeeding
- Depression
- Postpartum hemorrhage may occur soon after delivery but may occur up to 6 weeks later.

At your checkups, your health care provider can help spot and treat health conditions. Postpartum care is important because new moms are at risk of serious and sometimes life-threatening health complications in the days and weeks after giving birth.

Chapter 2

Realities of Post-partum

- ***Backaches and Headaches.***

Some new mothers experience headaches after they have a baby.This can be caused by the shifting hormones in your body as it returns to normal. Lack of sleep and the stress of being a new mother can also cause headaches.

Breastfeeding and the extra weight of full breasts can contribute to backaches. Be sure to wear a good, supportive bra. Pay attention to how you sleep, hold, carry, and feed your baby. For example, try to use a baby carrier or a sling instead of carrying your baby in his or her car seat. See if there are different ways you can sit or use pillows as props to relieve pressure on your neck and back. You can try putting heat on the muscles to help them relax or take a warm bath. You can also take some Ibuprofen to help with the pain. If your headache doesn't get better with Ibuprofen, call your provider.

- ***Alopecia***.

Each of the hairs on our head goes through 2 phases: a growing phase, which may last for several years, followed by a much shorter resting phase. After the resting phase, hair falls out and is replaced by new growth.

The body experiences soaring estrogen and progesterone levels during pregnancy, which causes hair to remain in an ongoing stage of growth, creating thicker, more lustrous strands. Then your hormones level out in the months following childbirth. Hair remains in this 'resting' stage for approximately three months before it falls out and new growth shows itself, typically the regrowth is in the form of baby bangs appearing along the hairline.

If you're finding a surplus of strands on your pillow or clogging the shower drain, you're not imagining things. When you haven't just had a baby, losing about 80 hairs per day is normal, but new moms shed about 400 hairs per day. By six months postpartum, the hair loss should slow to pre-pregnancy amounts.

If you feel the shedding is not slowing down, chances are good that there are other health issues at play. Pregnancy can change your level of ferritin (a blood cell protein that helps your body store iron) and can put your thyroid out of whack, so make sure to tell your doctor that you've noticed a lot of hair loss, and ask to have blood tests done to check both.

- ***Vaginal Soreness and Perineum Pain.***

If you had a vaginal tear and stitches, vaginal tissue has a great blood supply and will heal quickly.It can be very painful for the first week or two. Keep the area clean and squirt with warm water after you use the bathroom each time. Alternating ice packs with warm tub soaks will help with the pain and the healing process.It is best to refrain from sexual intercourse until the area is pain free.If you are continuing to experience pain at six weeks postpartum, your provider should check to make sure there is not a problem with the healing process.

The perineum is the area between your vagina and rectum. It stretches and may tear during labor and vaginal birth. It's often sore after giving birth, and it may be more sore if you have an episiotomy. This is a cut made at the opening of the vagina to help let your baby out.

What you can do:

- Do Kegel exercises. These exercises strengthen the muscles in the pelvic area. To do Kegel exercises, squeeze the muscles that you use to stop yourself from passing urine (peeing). Hold the muscles tight for 10 seconds and then release. Try to do this at least 10 times in a row, three times a day.

- Put a cold pack on your perineum. Use ice wrapped in a towel. Or you can buy cold packs that you freeze in your freezer.
- Sit on a pillow or a donut-shaped cushion.
- Soak in a warm bath.
- Wipe from front to back after going to the bathroom. This can help prevent infection as your episiotomy heals.
- Ask your provider about pain medicine.

- ***Hemorrhoids and Constipation.***

Hemorrhoids are varicose veins that develop in the rectal area.

Many women may develop a hemorrhoid during pregnancy or birth
because of the added pressure in your bottom. Hemorrhoids are painful, swollen veins in and around the anus that may hurt or bleed. Hemorrhoids are common during and after pregnancy.Hemorrhoids can be painful and itchy but usually go away within a few weeks of delivery

What you can do:

- Soak in a warm bath.
- Ask your provider about using an over-the-counter spray or cream for pain.
- Eat foods that are high in fiber, such as fruits, vegetables and whole-grain breads and cereals.
- Drink lots of water.

- Try not to strain when you're having a bowel movement (pooping).
- Witch hazel pads are usually recommended.
- Heat AND cold are usually helpful too. You might try alternating ice packs with soaking in a tub of very warm water.
- Your provider can also recommend medicine that has a numbing effect and/or prescribe a steroid medication that will decrease the swelling.

Constipation is when you don't have bowel movements, you don't have them often or your stools (poop) are hard to pass. You also may have painful gas. This may happen for a few days after you give birth.

Constipation is a common and usually short-lived problem that can

occur after delivery. It will definitely not help with the hemorrhoids.
Adding fiber (such as fruits, vegetables and whole grains) to your diet and trying an over-the-counter stool softener such as Colace or glycerine suppositories can help prevent constipation. Drinking lots of water can help too.

- ***Urinary problems and Sweating.***

During pregnancy and childbirth, the pelvic floor muscles, nerves and ligaments may get stretched and injured. In the first few days after giving birth, you may feel pain or burning when you urinate (pee). Or you may try to urinate but find that you can't. Sometimes you may not be able to stop urinating this is called stress incontinence.

What you can do for pain, burning or if you have trouble urinating:

- Drink lots of water.
- Run water in the sink when you go to the bathroom.
- Soak in a warm bath.
- If the pain continues, tell your provider.

What you can do for incontinence:
Do Kegel exercises to strengthen your pelvic muscles.

How to do Kegel Exercises

To find the correct muscles, try to stop the flow of urine while you
are peeing. The muscles you squeeze are the pelvic floor muscles.
Once you learn to do this exercise, do not do it while peeing.

To make these muscles stronger, squeeze and contract, then hold them for a few seconds. Repeat the process 10 times in a session. As the muscles become stronger, hold them longer. It's a good idea for women to do kegel exercises several times every day. You can do them anywhere.

Sweating happens often to new moms, especially at night. It's caused by all the changing hormones in your body after pregnancy.
What you can do:

- Sleep on a towel to help keep your sheets and pillow dry.
- Don't use too many blankets or wear warm clothes to bed.

- ***Weight problems and Skin changes.*** You lose about 10 pounds (4.536kg) right away after giving birth and a little more within the first week. This is a great time to get to a healthy weight, no matter how much you weighed before you got pregnant. Eating healthy and being active every day helps boost your energy level and can make you feel better. If you're at a healthy weight, you're less likely to have health conditions, like diabetes and high blood pressure, than if you're over- or underweight. And just in case you get pregnant again, or if you're planning to have another baby sometime in the future, it's best to be at a healthy weight before your next pregnancy.

What you can do:

- Talk to your provider about your weight. If you were overweight before pregnancy, you may want to lose more weight than you gained during pregnancy.
- Eat healthy foods. Limit sweets and foods with a lot of fat.
- Drink lots of water.
- Ask your provider about being active, especially if you've had a c-section. Begin slowly and increase your activity over time. Walking and swimming are great activities for new moms. Do something active every day.
- Breastfeed your baby. Breastfeeding helps you burn calories. This can help you lose the weight you gained

during pregnancy faster than if you weren't breastfeeding.

- Don't try to lose too much weight too fast. Your body needs nutrients from food to heal. If you're breastfeeding, losing weight too fast can reduce your milk supply.
- Don't feel badly if you don't lose the weight as quickly as you'd like. It takes time for your body and your belly to get back in shape. Staying fit over time is more important than getting in shape right after giving birth.

You may have Skin problems such as stretch marks on your belly where your skin stretched during pregnancy. Some women also get them on their thighs, hips and bottom. They may not disappear after giving birth, but they do fade over time.

Extra skin, stretch marks, changing breast sizes, changing shoe sizes, different hair texture, varicose veins, consider these a badge of courage.

What you can do:

Use creams or lotions on your skin. They don't make stretch marks go away, but they can help reduce itching that comes with stretch marks.

- ***Breast Engorgement and Sore Nipples.***

This is when your breasts swell as they fill with milk. It usually happens a few days after giving birth. Your breasts may feel tender and sore. The discomfort usually goes away once you start breastfeeding regularly. If you're not breastfeeding, it may last until your breasts stop making milk, usually within a few days.

What you can do:

- Breastfeed your baby. Try not to miss a feeding or go a long time between feedings. Don't skip night feedings.
- Before you breastfeed your baby, express a small amount of milk from your breast with a breast pump or by hand.
- Take a warm shower or lay warm towels on your breasts to help your milk flow. If your engorgement is really painful, put cold packs on your breasts.
- If your breasts are leaking between feedings, wear nursing pads in your bra so your clothes don't get wet.

- Tell your provider if your breasts stay swollen and are painful.
- If you're not planning to breastfeed, wear a firm, supportive bra (like a sports bra).

Sore Nipple: If you're breastfeeding, you may have sore nipple during the first few days, especially if your nipples crack.

What you can do:

- Talk to your provider or a lactation consultant to be sure your baby is latching on to your breast the right way. A lactation consultant is a person trained to help women breastfeed, even women who have breastfeeding problems. Latching on is when your baby's mouth is securely attached to (placed around) your nipple.

- Ask your provider about cream to put on your nipples.
- After breastfeeding, massage some breast milk onto your nipples. Let your breasts air dry.

- ***Vaginal Discharge***

After your baby is born, your body gets rid of the blood and tissue that was inside your uterus. This is called vaginal discharge or lochia. For the first few days, it's heavy, bright red and may contain blood clots. Over time, the flow gets less and lighter in color. You may have discharge for a few weeks or even for a month or more.

What you can do:

Use sanitary pads until the discharge stops.

- ***Cesarean Section and Tiredness after Childbirth***

Cesarean birth (also called c-section) is surgery in which your baby is born through a cut that your provider makes in your belly and uterus. A c-section is major surgery, so it may take a while for you to recover. You may be really tired for the first few days or weeks after a c-section because you lost blood during the surgery. The incision (cut) on your belly may be sore. A number of nerves were cut during the procedure and will take time to repair. It can take up to six months for all of the nerves in the abdominal area to heal completely. Some women continue to experience numbness, tingling and odd shooting pains around their scar for months after delivery.

What you can do:

- Ask your provider for pain medicine. Check with him before you take any medicine for pain.
- Ask your partner, family and friends to help you with the baby and around the house.
- Get rest when you can. Sleep when your baby sleeps, even when he naps during the day.
- Don't lift from a squatting position. Don't lift anything heavier than your baby.
- Support your belly with pillows when you're breastfeeding.
- Drink plenty of water to help replace fluids in your body.

You may have lost blood during labor and birth. This can make your body tired. And your baby probably doesn't let you sleep all night!

What you can do:

- Sleep when your baby sleeps, even when he naps during the day.
- Eat healthy foods, like fruits, vegetables, whole-grain breads and pasta, and lean meat and chicken. Limit sweets and foods with a lot of fat.
- Ask your partner, family and friends for help with the baby and around the house.
- Limit visitors. You'll have plenty of time for family and friends to meet your new baby when you're feeling rested.

Chapter 3

Baby Blues versus Post-partum Depression.

Baby blues (also called postpartum blues) are feelings of sadness a woman may have in the first few days after having a baby. Baby blues can happen 2 to 3 days after you have your baby and can last up to 2 weeks. They usually go away on their own, and you don't need any treatment.

Postpartum depression (also called PPD) is a kind of depression that some women get after having a baby. It's strong feelings of sadness, anxiety (worry) and tiredness that last for a long time after giving birth. These feelings can make it hard for you to take care of yourself and your baby. PPD is a medical condition that needs treatment to get better. It's the most common complication for women who have just had a baby.

Having a baby is a really big deal.Mothers often have a lot of different
feelings and emotions in the weeks and months after they give birth.
These feelings can change often and go from happy to sad to worried
to scared and back again. Mothers may find that things affect them
more now than they did before.
Most mothers may experience the "baby blues".They may feel sad and
cry easily for a little while after they have a baby. Some mothers
experience much stronger feelings.These moms may have postpartum

depression. Postpartum depression happens more than most women know. In fact, one out of every ten new mothers has postpartum depression.
Postpartum depression can be very serious and prevent you from caring for yourself and your baby.Talk to your healthcare provider if you feel sad or depressed.

What you can do about the baby blues:

- Get as much sleep as you can.
- Don't drink alcohol, use street drugs or use harmful drugs. All of these can affect your mood and make you feel worse. And they can make it hard for you to take care of your baby.

- Ask for help from your partner, family and friends. Tell them exactly what they can do for you.
- Take time for yourself. Ask someone you trust to watch your baby so you can get out of the house.
- Connect with other new moms. Ask your provider to help you find a support group of new moms.
- If you have sad feelings that last longer than 2 weeks, tell your health care provider.

What you can do about postpartum depression:

- If you think you have PPD, tell your provider.
- Learn about risk factors for PPD and signs and symptoms of PPD.

- Ask your provider about treatment for PPD.
- If you're worried about hurting yourself or your baby, call emergency services (911) right away.

Chapter 4

Adjusting to Motherhood

Your Family:

A woman's relationship with her mother and other family members may feel especially important after the birth of a baby. Having a baby can bring up many different feelings. Sometimes having help is good and sometimes it can be hard. It can be even more complicated when in-laws are involved! It can be wonderful to get the advice of someone who has been through the same things you are going through and who may be able to share helpful tips. It can also be stressful, especially if this advice is unwanted or makes you feel like you don't know what you are doing.

Have visitors? Try making a list of chores and errands that need to be done. For example, have them do a load of laundry, make a meal that can be frozen, or play games with an older child. Think about what you need and ask for it. Grab a nap.

If you get advice that is different from what you think is right, it's okay to ask your health care provider or other friends for a second opinion. When in doubt, trust your instincts.

Your Partner:

Men have health and emotional needs too. Some dads may feel a lot of stress after the birth of a baby. They may need to do more around the house and take care of other children. Some feel worried about money. Many dads are tired too. The birth of a baby can be an event that can bring two people closer together. It can also make them very stressed out! Dads need to ask for help too.

Both you and your partner are getting used to having a baby around. Your partner may be just as stressed and nervous about being a parent as you are. Rely on each other to figure things out.

What you can do:

- Learn about taking care of your baby together. Read baby-care books and go to baby-care classes.
- Let your partner help with the baby. Don't try to do everything yourself.

- Talk to each other. Talking about your feelings can help keep you from feeling hurt and frustrated.
- Make time for just the two of you. Go for a walk or out to dinner. Ask someone you trust to take care of the baby for an hour or two.
- Tell your partner what your provider says about how long to wait to have sex again. Ask your provider to talk to your partner, if you think that's helpful.

Work and School:

It may be hard for you to leave your baby with a caregiver all day, even if it's a family member or a close friend. It also may be hard to find a caregiver you trust. You and your partner may disagree about what type of child care is best for your baby. You may be upset that you can't stay home with your baby all the time.

What you can do:

- Talk to your partner about child care. Figure out how much you can spend and what kind of care you want. For example, you can have a caregiver come to your home to take care of your baby. Or you can take your baby to a child care center.
- Ask friends and family about child care they use. Maybe you can use the same person or service.
- If you're using a child care center, ask for names and phone numbers of people who use the center. Call to ask how they feel about the center's care.

- Ask your boss if you can ease back into work. Maybe you can work a few hours a day at first, or just a few days a week.

Connect with Other Moms:

No one knows what you're going through as well as someone who is going through it too.Link up with other moms! Many communities and churches have groups. Check for groups at the library, online, and at your pediatrician's office.

Don't be afraid to ask for help if you are:

• Feeling really, really tired almost all the time

• Feeling really worried

• Crying all the time

• Not being able to sleep, even when the baby is asleep
• Having scary thoughts
• Feeling guilty
• Having a change in appetite
• Being so tired and worried that you can't care for the baby
• Not being able to feel happy or to enjoy simple things, like
reading a good magazine or catching up with a friend.

Overwhelmed and Stressed:

Your baby didn't come with a set of instructions. You may feel overwhelmed trying to take care of her. Taking care of a baby is a lot to think about.

What you can do:

- Tell your partner how you feel. Let your partner help take care of the baby.
- Ask your friends and family for help. Tell them exactly what they can do for you, like going grocery shopping or making meals.
- Find a support group of new moms. A support group is a group of people who have the same kinds of concerns. They meet together to try to help each other. Ask your provider to help you find a support group of new moms near where you live. Or look for a support group online.
- Eat healthy foods and do something active every day.
- Don't smoke, drink alcohol or use harmful drugs. All of these things are bad for you and can make it hard for you to handle stress.

Chapter 5

Coping with body changes.

The reality is pregnancy changes our bodies (and brains) in a variety of ways, and having realistic expectations about that is important. Our skin stretches, some of us experience abdominal muscle separation (diastasis recti), our hips widen, our bones get bigger, our breasts change density and shape, and our feet grow.
A healthy weight gain during pregnancy is an average of 25 to 35 pounds. Here is where that weight comes from:

- Additional 2 pounds of the uterus as it grows
- Placenta weights 1.5 pounds
- Fluid volume is 4 pounds

- Breast tissue increases an additional 2 pounds
- Blood volume adds 4 pounds
- There are 7 pounds of nutrients
- 2 pounds of amniotic fluid
- An average of 7.5 pounds for the baby.

And though this is all supposed to happen, our bodies have to expand and shift in profound ways to develop, make room for and grow another human, many of us can't help but feel frustrated, insecure and even ashamed about the way our bodies look after we give birth.

Becoming a mom, like any transition in life, can be hard on the body and the mind. The postpartum period comes with so many unknowns, and it may feel like you don't have any control over your body and perhaps in your new role as a mom, but please try to remember: ***you have the power to make a healthy shift in your mindset and life.***

Whether you believe it or not, your body doesn't need to conform to unrealistic standards. It is amazing and beautiful and unique, and I want to help you learn to accept, honor and love it.

Contributors to Postpartum Body Shame.

- *Media & Cultural Expectations*

We are constantly being bombarded by cultural expectations of how our bodies should look. Take a second to scroll through your social media feed, peruse any pop culture website or magazine, or think about all the products that exist to help you "lose weight quickly." Society places an insane emphasis on thinness and physical appearance, the "perfect body."

Of course, everyone knows a woman must gain weight in order to grow a healthy baby, so expectant women are exempt from the expectation of thinness. But sadly, that respite doesn't last long after the baby is born. Indeed, we're somehow led to believe that we should be able to quickly lose the baby weight and fit back into our pre-pregnancy wardrobe.
This idea is unrealistic, highly damaging and outrightly dangerous, as it leads so many new moms to feel like failures and like less versions of their former selves. For some new moms, it can trigger deep

feelings of disgust and self-loathing every time they look in the mirror, and, in certain circumstances, may also lead to postpartum depression.

- ***Feelings of Insecurity, Loss and Uncertainty in Transition to New Motherhood.***

The negative feelings you may experience about your postpartum body could be about more than just your physical appearance. The loss of a woman's pre-baby body, the body you've gotten used to and known since becoming a woman is tangible, visible evidence and a reminder that her life and identity has changed significantly, and that can feel incredibly scary, isolating and overwhelming.

According to the NYT, the body is symbolic. ***"For many new mothers, a***

struggle with body image is intertwined with the desire to reclaim parts of themselves that have been pushed aside by the physical and emotional demands of new parenthood. Have compassion for yourself as you go through this identity transition, and be as gentle with your own body as you are with your baby's."

More often than not, a baby can change your relationship with your partner. You may feel less romantic, more resentful and less connected emotionally and physically.

There's also the loss in autonomy and independence. After a baby arrives, a woman's time doesn't truly belong to her anymore, her baby's schedule likely dictates her own. Not to mention the major changes, often losses, many women experience in their careers.

- ***History of Disordered Eating and Distorted Body Image.***

A strong predictor of negative body image after pregnancy, is negative body image before pregnancy, as well as a history of disordered eating.
In addition, for many women who have worked hard to gain control over an eating disorder or unhealthy body image concerns, the hyper-focus on one's body and weight during pregnancy, as well as the necessary pregnancy weight-gain, may trigger a relapse.

Protective Measures to Take During Pregnancy.

- **Have Realistic Expectations.**

Our bodies don't miraculously transform back to their pre-baby versions once we give birth, this is a fact we just have to accept. Understand that this is normal and healthy. Rather than focusing on appearance, focus on how you feel instead.

- **Change your Wardrobe**

You will likely go through an awkward period of not knowing what to wear. While investing in pieces that you see as temporary might not feel like a great use of money, it's super important to have some nice things to wear that make you feel comfortable and confident.

- **Mindfulness Activities**

If you find yourself so preoccupied with your weight gain, or fear about not being able to lose the weight after you have the baby, try some deep breathing techniques and mindfulness exercises. Journaling and writing about your concerns may also be a good way to let them out.

- **Speak Up**

People are fascinated by pregnant women, it's like seeing alien species up close and in real life.

If people around you, friends, family, strangers, etc. are constantly talking about or focused on your body and it's making you uncomfortable, don't be afraid to tell them to stop.

- **Ask for Help**

If these tips aren't working for you and you are still worried about how you might feel about your body after you give birth, don't be ashamed to seek professional help. Be proactive!

How to Love, Honor and Appreciate your Post-Partum Body.

- **Ditch the scale.**

The only reason you need a scale is to weigh luggage, and no one's going anywhere these days. Your health care provider will weigh you at your postnatal visits, and if there's a problem, he/she will tell you.

- **Stop body-checking.**

Spending time in front of the mirror judging and berating yourself is a huge waste of time and energy.

- **Toss out the magazines.**

It's not helpful or fair to compare yourself to the models and feel badly that your postpartum body doesn't look like theirs. Not to mention, they also may be doing things to lose weight that aren't healthy skipping meals, taking diet pills, etc. If you want to change your body, do it to be healthier, feel stronger, and have a better mindset mentally and physically. Skinny doesn't equal healthy.

- **Quit the Social Media Comparison Game.**

Social media is a tricky platform that really complicates the issue: on the one hand, many moms and influencers claim to portray a more "realistic" representation of motherhood and of what the postpartum body looks like.

As women share their postpartum journey, Instagram, for instance, becomes a space where women can relate, feel less alone in their struggles, and build a strong sense of community with fellow new moms. But on the other hand, it can be difficult to differentiate sponsored content from "regular" content, and the "realistic" portrayal of motherhood is still often curated, filtered and beautified. Not to mention, in most cases, it doesn't quite reflect the experience most of us have in those early days/weeks/months of postpartum, which is normal, just like pregnancy, every mom's postpartum journey is unique.

Remember, social media, these days, is often just another advertising platform that reaches directly in your living room, while you are nursing your baby or trying to take a nap. You don't know what really goes on behind those filtered, “trying not to look posed, but posed” images. That mama may also be experiencing some negative feelings about her changes, but may be putting on a face for the camera and the sake of her grid.

- **Talk to yourself the way you’d want your child to talk to him/herself.**

Here’s a good piece of advice from an article in the NYT: “If you ever berate yourself, stop and ask whether you would want your child to speak to herself that way. Use your relationship with your body image as an indicator that you may need to learn how to be less critical and more patient with yourself and others.”

- **Switch your frame of mind.**

When you find yourself feeling upset about or ashamed of your body, do your best to try to change your thinking.

Your belly is larger because you brought a baby into the world. Now that's a superpower, mama!
The marks on your skin, stretch marks, dark spots, etc., are badges of honor you can wear proudly; you did the hard work of growing and birthing a baby. You're incredible!

- **Health first.**

When you do start up with an exercise or nutrition program, make sure to focus on

health not weight loss and set healthy and realistic goals for yourself.
Also, if you've had any abdominal separation (diastasis recti), you'll want to check with your doctor before beginning a program, and seek the help of a physical therapist or find an exercise program that's well versed in the unique needs of postpartum women.

- **Seek professional help.**

If you are struggling to manage your negative feelings about your body and it's preventing you from caring for yourself, your baby and living your life, it's time to seek professional help from a therapist and/or a dietician well-versed in postpartum health and body image concerns.

Chapter 6

Functioning as a Family Unit

As overlooked as a Mother's health is after delivery, it is very much important as the child to take good care of the Mother's health. Most often, mothers lack the capacity to take care of themselves after delivery. As a family or friend, a new mom needs all the help she can get, from chores to taking care of the home, meals, newborn and even herself.
Here are some of the things you can do to ensure her health is being cared for:

- **Make it about her, not the baby.**

That means showing up prepared to listen and making the conversation about her every single time. You shouldn't be doing more talking than she is, either. Make it safe for her to share any feelings that she is having, even if they don't make much sense.

- **Stop trying to solve her problems.** We often try to cheer up others by disputing their emotions. But comments like "What are you talking about? You're a great mom!" are actually counterproductive. It won't make her feel like a great mom, Instead, it invalidates her feelings and can even trigger feelings of guilt. Instead, echo the mother's concerns with statements like "It sounds like you're really worried" or "That must be really hard." If you've experienced anxiety or depression before, even unrelated to pregnancy, offer up your own story to show that you understand what she is going through. Because women often feel alone when experiencing depression, it can be helpful to hear other women share their experiences.

- **Celebrate her successes.**

Celebrate her successes, no matter how little, find a fun way to celebrate with her.

- **Offer to go to doctor's appointments with her.**

This isn't about keeping her company; it's about being her advocate. She will likely have a team of practitioners to follow up with during the first year, but these postnatal checkups are usually focused on the baby, so Mom's needs and concerns could get overlooked. Ask if you can tag along to those appointments if her partner can't attend. This isn't to undermine her, but to bring up anything that feels off for her, in case the doctor doesn't ask.

- **Quit asking what you can do and just start doing it**

It may be well intentioned, but saying "If you need anything at all, I'm here" to a sleep-deprived and depressed mother isn't very helpful. It puts the onus on her to figure out what she needs, which she may be struggling to understand. Be specific and direct in the help you offer. If she isn't sleeping when she gets the chance (a warning sign of PPD), ask if you can take the baby off her hands while she naps, showers or goes somewhere for a few hours. If there's an older child in the picture, offer to do daycare pickup or drop-off. And, because she may not be eating regularly, arrive with her favourite food when you visit.

Conclusion

The postpartum period can be hard both physically and emotionally.
If you're a new mom and you can't remember if you even brushed your teeth this morning, welcome to postpartum life. Ask just about any mom about the days, weeks, and months after having a baby, and you're sure to get a similar response. Something like, "I'm really tired." Having a baby takes a toll on a mom's body, mind, and spirit. It's not all bad and exhausting, but it's not all unicorns and rainbows either. Not for every woman all the time, anyway. Unfortunately, the postpartum period (which can impact women for up to a year after birth) is just not simple, and assuming that it is leaves mom to fend for herself.

That is why it is very important and critical for you as a mom and also as a care giver, to focus on Mama's health as much as you do the newborn.
During the healing process, make sure your body is ready before resuming certain physical activities. If you had an episiotomy, vaginal tear, or cesarean delivery during birth, the time before you can resume certain activities may vary.
By the time you're ready for your post-birth exam 6 to 8 weeks after delivery, you may start to feel more like yourself physically.

But if at any time after leaving the hospital your bleeding becomes heavier, you experience a fever over 100.4°F (38°C), or you see a pus-like discharge coming from one of your incisions, call your doctor.

It never hurts to get some peace of mind with any questions or concerns you may have.
Doctors generally advise to wait about 6 weeks after a vaginal birth, and 8 weeks after a cesarean birth, before having sexual intercourse.

Hormone changes during pregnancy and the act of giving birth itself might make sex uncomfortable at first.

Also be aware that immediately following childbirth and before your menstrual cycle resumes, you're especially likely to get pregnant again.

Make sure you've chosen a method of birth control before having sex with a partner capable of getting you pregnant.

If you're breastfeeding, you may find yourself feeling hungry often. This indicates that you need to consume extra calories to make up for the calories lost to making milk for your baby.

According to the Centers for Disease Control and Prevention (CDC)Trusted Source, you'll want to eat approximately 2,300 to 2,500 calories per day. This will depend on your body, activity levels, and other factors. Discuss your caloric needs with your doctor.

Continue taking your prenatal vitamins while you breastfeed. Drinking plenty of water is also vital.

Also continue to restrict the substances you avoided during pregnancy, in particular:

- alcohol
- caffeine
- high mercury fish, such as tuna and swordfish

While you don't have to avoid alcohol or caffeine completely, be mindful of the amount you consume and the timing of your consumption. This will help keep baby from being exposed to these potentially harmful substances.

You may want to jump right into an eating plan that will restore your "pre-baby body." But the most important thing you can do for the first few weeks after childbirth is to heal and restore the vitamins and minerals you may have lost during delivery.

While in the hospital, your baby's hearing and eyesight will also be tested. Your baby will also be tested for their blood type. Some states have laws or recommendations that mandate babies receive certain vaccines or medications before they leave the hospital.

The rest of baby's experience in the hospital will depend on their birth weight and how they're doing after birth.

Some babies who aren't considered full term (born before 37 weeks) or are born with a low birth weight are kept for observation in a neonatal intensive care unit (NICU) to ensure that they can adjust to life after the womb.

Newborn jaundice, which involves a yellowing of the skin, is fairly common. Around 60 percent of newborn babies experience jaundice.

Babies with jaundice will need to be treated in an incubator.

Before you leave the hospital, you'll need to make an appointment with a pediatrician outside the hospital to weigh and examine baby. This 1-week appointment is standard practice.

This book offers about 60% knowledge you need to achieve a healthy postpartum journey, the 40% rest on your choice and ability to make it happen.
Sending hugs and love to you Moms!

My Firm Resolve:

www.ingramcontent.com/pod-product-compliance
Lightning Source LLC
LaVergne TN
LVHW010459160826
845677LV00012B/2558

* 9 7 9 8 8 4 8 8 5 3 8 2 7 *